YOUR KNOWLEDGE HAS \

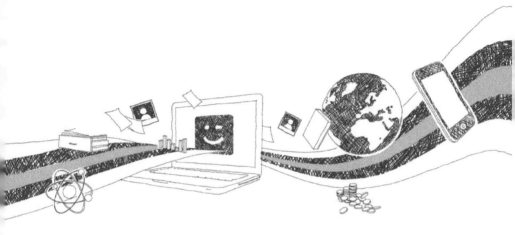

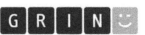

Bibliographic information published by the German National Library:

The German National Library lists this publication in the National Bibliography; detailed bibliographic data are available on the Internet at http://dnb.dnb.de .

Imprint:

Copyright © 2016 GRIN Verlag, Open Publishing GmbH
Print and binding: Books on Demand GmbH, Norderstedt Germany
ISBN: 9783668335295

This book at GRIN:

http://www.grin.com/en/e-book/341580/in-silico-modeling-and-identification-of-novel-epitopes-based-vaccine-of

Marwa Osman, et al.

In Silico Modeling and Identification of Novel Epitopes-based Vaccine of M polyprotein (Gn/Gc) against Schmallenberg Virus for Ruminants

GRIN Publishing

GRIN - Your knowledge has value

Since its foundation in 1998, GRIN has specialized in publishing academic texts by students, college teachers and other academics as e-book and printed book. The website www.grin.com is an ideal platform for presenting term papers, final papers, scientific essays, dissertations and specialist books.

Visit us on the internet:

http://www.grin.com/

http://www.facebook.com/grincom

http://www.twitter.com/grin_com

In Silico Modeling and Identification of Novel Epitopes based Vaccine of M polyprotein (Gn/Gc) against Schmallenberg Virus for Ruminants

Nesreen Abdelhamied Abdelrazig*, Marwa Mohamed Osman*, ,Ahmed Mohammed Adam, Neema Esmat Mahmud, Israa Elawad Osman, Fatima Attaelfadail Awadelkareem , Ezdihar Elhadi ElAmin, , Afra Abd Elhamid Fadl Alla, Soada Ahmed Osman, Ahmed Abubakar Elsayed & Mohamed Ahmed Salih

Department of Biotechnology, Africa city of Technology- Khartoum, Sudan

*contributed equally

ABSTRACT

Schmallenberg (SBV) is a new virus of the Bunyaviridae family within the genus Orthobunyavirus. Viral infection causes mild clinical signs: fever, reduced milk production diarrhea and considerable economic loss. Unfortunately currently there is no treatment or vaccine for infected animals. We aimed to design peptide vaccine using Immunoinformatics approach to stimulate the immune system and reducing the potential negative effects of using live vaccines. In this study total of 47 strains of complete M polyprotein sequence (Gn/NSm/GC) and 61 strains of nonstructural protein in S segment (NSs) of Schmallenberg virus which chosen for this study were taken from NCBI. Potentially continuous B and T cell epitopes were predicted using tools from immune epitope data base analysis resource (IEDB-AR). We found that Gn and Gc regions of M polyprotein in SBV was clearly suitable and could be used for the preparation of immunological constructs. Our studies suggested that; B cell epitope $^{764}QQQACSS^{770}$ and CTL epitopes $^{251}YMYNKYFKL^{259}$, $^{46}SECCVKDDI^{54}$ and $^{234}IVYVFIPIF^{242}$ could be used as a potential vaccine candidate against SBV. We considered this study distinctive because no research ever dealt with peptide based vaccine on virulent strains of SBV using in silico approach.

Key words: Schmallenberg (SBV), ruminants, epitopes, overlapping & vaccine

Contents

INTRODUCTION

In 2011, in the German town of Schmallenberg a new virus of the *Bunyaviridae* family, a member of the Simbu serogroup within the genus *Orthobunyavirus* has been identified for first time, which was called later Schmallenberg virus (SBV)[1,2,3]. SBV genome consists of three segments of negative sense, single-stranded RNA the L (large), M (medium) and S (small) segments [4,5]. The L segment encodes the RNA dependent RNA polymerase; M segment encodes surface glycoproteins Gn and Gc which they form spikes on the virus particle and are essential for viral attachment and cell fusion, and nonstructural protein NSm. The S segment encodes nucleocapsid protein N and nonstructural protein NSs. NSs is considered a major virulence factor for orthobunyaviruses and has able to counteract host antiviral responses [6-8].

SBV affect mainly domestic and wild ruminants, such as cattle, sheep, goats, mouflon, moose, alpacas, buffalos, bison, and deer [9,10]. Moreover antibodies of virus were also found in Swedish dogs [11]. SBV is transmitted by an arthropod vector, principally *Culicoides* biting midges, while virus has also been identified in the semen of bulls but venereal transmission has not yet been demonstrated [12-14] Viral infection causes mild clinical signs in adult cattle fever, reduced milk production and diarrhea, but infection of susceptible pregnant animals can associated with abortions, stillbirths and malformations of the skeletal and central nervous system (CNS) in newborn ruminants [15-18].

After the initial detection the virus has been spread to at least 20 countries in Europe such as Netherlands, Belgium, United Kingdom, France, Italy, Spain, Poland and Ireland, 8,730 herds and flocks reported infected by May 2013 just in Western Europe. Furthermore, a high percentage of antibody-positive animals in some ruminants of the Zambezia Province in Mozambique were recorded [19-27].

Since the emergence of SBV in Europe, efforts was exerted to reduce the mortality and morbidity rats, one of the experimental vaccine, the trivalent vaccine against the Simbu serogroup viruses Akabane virus and Aino virus and the reovirus Chuzan, but this vaccine failed to provide prevention from SBV infection. However two commercial inactivated vaccines have already been granted a provisional marketing authorization in the United Kingdom and France, but highly efficacious and safe live vaccines are still not available[3, 28-31]. Antibodies specific for Simbu serogroup viruses frequently cross-react with more than one other member

3

of the two surface glycoproteins Gn and Gc and the viral polymerase complex composed of the polymerase L protein and the nucleoprotein N. This complex is responsible for the transcription and replication of the viruses that occur exclusively in the cytoplasm. Inside the virus particle, the viral genome is present as a ribonucleoprotein (RNP) associated with many copies of the nucleoprotein N and a few copies of the polymerase L. is serogroup [32, 33]. Since Akabane virus (AKAV) or Aino virus (AINOV) causes similar clinical signs to Schmallenberg virus [3]. Scientists found that vaccines against AKAV and AINOV, could potentially offer a tool for disease control until an SBV-specific vaccine is ready for use [3].

This study took a different direction by design peptide vaccine work to stimulate the immune system and reduce the potential negative effects of using live vaccines generally, based on *in silico* approach and computational methods.

Material and Methods

Protein Sequence Retrieval

The 47 strains of complete M polyprotein sequence (Gn/NSm/GC) and 61 strains of nonstructural protein in S segment (NSs) of Schmallenberg virus which chosen for this study were taken from NCBI database (http://www.ncbi.nlm.nih.gov) in FASTA format in May 2016. The Nonstructural protein (NSm) in M polyprotein was excluded from this study. The length of M polyprotein was found between 1391-1403 amino acids, Table (1) while the length of NSs protein was 91 amino acids. These strains were isolated from different geographical regions from Bos taurus (cattle), Ovis aries (sheep) and Capra hircus (goats) from 2011-2014, Table (2).

Retrieved Strains Phylogeny

The relationships of all retrieved strains of M polyprotein sequence were studied using phylogeny.fr online software (http://phylogeny.lirmm.fr/phylo_cgi/index.cgi) [34].

Table (1): M polyprotein of Schmallenburgvirus and its length

polyprotein	abbrivation	length
Glycoprotein Gn	Gn: G1	558-1342
Nonstructural protein	NSm	309-459
Glycoprotein Gc	Gc: G2	23-308

Table (2): retrieved sequences with their hosts and area of collection

M Polyprotein Accession No.	Date of Collection	Host	Country	NSs Protein Accession No.	Date of Collection	Host	Country
H2AM12.1	2011	Cattle	Germany	H2AM14.1	2011	Cattle	Germany
AGC93536.1	2012	Cattle	Germany	AGU16234.1	2011	Sheep	Netherlands
AGC93535.1	2012	Cattle	Germany	AGU16238.1	2011	Cattle	Netherlands
AGC93534.1	2012	Sheep	Germany	AKA63342.1	2014	Cattle	Germany
AGC93533.1	2012	Sheep	Germany	AKA63340.1	2014	Cattle	Germany
AGC93532.1	2012	Sheep	Germany	AKA63338.1	2014	Cattle	Germany
AGC93531.1	2012	Cattle	Germany	AKA63336.1	2012	Cattle	Germany
AGC93530.1	2012	Cattle	Germany	AKA63334.1	2012	Cattle	Germany

Accession	Year	Host	Country	Accession	Year	Host	Country
AGC93529.1	2012	Sheep	Germany	AKA63332.1	2012	Cattle	Germany
AGC93528.1	2012	Goat	Germany	AGD94641.1	2012	Sheep	Belgium
AGC93527.1	2012	Goat	Germany	AGD94639.1	2012	Sheep	Belgium
AGC93526.1	2012	Sheep	Germany	AGD94637.1	2012	Sheep	Belgium
AGC93525.1	2012	Sheep	Germany	AGD94635.1	2012	Sheep	Belgium
AGC93524.1	2012	Sheep	Germany	AGD94633.1	2012	Sheep	Belgium
AGC93523.1	2012	Sheep	Germany	AGD94631.1	2012	Sheep	Belgium
AGC93522.1	2012	Sheep	Germany	CCF55032.1	2011	Cattle	Germany
AGC93521.1	2012	Sheep	Germany	AGC84163.1	2011	Unknown	Germany
AGC93520.1	2012	Sheep	Germany	ANJ16630.1	2012	Sheep	Belgium
AGC93519.1	2012	Sheep	Germany	ANJ16628.1	2012	Sheep	Belgium
AGC93518.1	2012	Sheep	Germany	ANJ16626.1	2012	Sheep	Belgium
AGC93517.1	2012	Sheep	Germany	ANJ16624.1	2011	Sheep	Belgium
AGC93516.1	2012	Sheep	Germany	ANJ16620.1	2012	Sheep	Belgium
AGC93515.1	2012	Sheep	Germany	ANJ16618.1	2012	Sheep	Belgium
AGC93514.1	2011	Sheep	Germany	ANJ16610.1	2012	Sheep	Belgium
AGU16236.1	2011	Cattle	Netherlands	ANJ16608.1	2012	Sheep	Belgium
AGU16232.1	2011	Cattle	Netherlands	ANJ16602.1	2013	Sheep	Belgium
AKA63348.1	2014	Cattle	Germany	ANJ16600.1	2012	Sheep	Belgium
AKA63347.1	2014	Cattle	Germany	ANJ16598.1	2012	Sheep	Belgium
AKA63346.1	2014	Cattle	Germany	ANJ16596.1	2012	Sheep	Belgium

Accession	Year	Host	Country	Accession	Year	Host	Country
AKA63345.1	2012	Cattle	Germany	ANJ16594.1	2012	Sheep	Belgium
AKA63344.1	2012	Cattle	Germany	ANJ16592.1	2013	Sheep	Belgium
AKA63343.1	2012	Cattle	Germany	ANJ16590.1	2012	Sheep	Belgium
CCF55030.1	2011	Cattle	Germany	ANJ16588.1	2011	Sheep	Belgium
AGC84161.1	2011	Unknown	Germany	ANJ16586.1	2013	Sheep	Belgium
AGD94648.1	2012	Sheep	Belgium	ANJ16584.1	2012	Sheep	Belgium
AGD94647.1	2012	Sheep	Belgium	ANJ16582.1	2012	Sheep	Belgium
AGD94646.1	2012	Sheep	Belgium	ANJ16580.1	2012	Sheep	Belgium
AGD94644.1	2012	Sheep	Belgium	ANJ16578.1	2012	Sheep	Belgium
AGD94643.1	2012	Sheep	Belgium	ANJ16576.1	2012	Sheep	Belgium
AGD94642.1	2012	Sheep	Belgium	ANJ16574.1	2012	Sheep	Belgium
AIP98333.1	2012	Cattle	Liechtenstein	ANJ16572.1	2012	Sheep	Belgium
AIP98332.1	2012	Cattle	Liechtenstein	ANJ16570.1	2012	Sheep	Belgium
AIP98331.1	2012	Cattle	Liechtenstein	ANJ16568.1	2011	Sheep	Belgium
AIP98330.1	2012	Cattle	Switzerland	ANJ16566.1	2012	Sheep	Belgium
AIP98329.1	2012	Cattle	Switzerland	ANJ16564.1	2012	Sheep	Belgium
AIP98327.1	2012	Cattle	Switzerland	ANJ16562.1	2012	Sheep	Belgium
AIP98328.1	2012	Cattle	Switzerland	ANJ16560.1	2012	Sheep	Belgium
				ANJ16558.1	2012	Sheep	Belgium
				ANJ16556.1	2013	Sheep	Belgium
				ANJ16554.1	2013	Sheep	Belgium

ANJ16552.1	2012	Sheep	Belgium
ANJ16550.1	2012	Sheep	Belgium
ANJ16548.1	2012	Sheep	Belgium
ANJ16546.1	2012	Sheep	Belgium
ANJ16544.1	2012	Sheep	Belgium
ANJ16542.1	2012	Sheep	Belgium
ANJ16540.1	2012	Sheep	Belgium
ANJ16538.1	2012	Sheep	Belgium
ANJ16536.1	2012	Sheep	Belgium
ANJ16534.1	2012	Sheep	Belgium
ANJ16532.1	2012	Sheep	Belgium

Identification of Conserved Regions

The retrieved sequences were subjected to multiple sequence alignment (MSA) using BioEdit software [35] to obtain conserved regions with conservancy percentage (100%). These conserved regions were used for B and T Cells predictions. The conservancy across antigen tool (http://tools.iedb.org/tools/conservancy/iedb_input) [36] was applied for more confirmation.

Epitope Prediction

IEDB-AR (http://www.iedb.org/) [37] was used for searching and exporting immune epitopes that could activate B and T cells.

B cell Epitope Prediction

For B cell epitopes prediction, four algorithms (http://tools.iedb.org/bcell/) were used: Bepipred linear epitope prediction method was used using hidden Markov model with default threshold 0.35 [38]. Scales with default threshold values for Emini surface accessibility prediction (1.000) [39], Kolaskar and Tongaonkar Antigenicity (1.039/1.029 in M polyprotein /NSs protein) [40] and Parker Hydrophilicity prediction (0.999/0.353 in M polyprotein /NSs protein) [41] tools were interpreted to choose between epitopes. Chou and Fasman Beta turn prediction method with default thresholds (0.981/0.986. 353 in M polyprotein/ NSs protein) [42] was used for more confirmation. Epitopes which passed these tests were predicted as B cell epitope.

T cell Epitope Prediction

For T cell epitopes, MHC I binding prediction tools (http://tools.iedb.org/mhci/) were applied to predict Cytotoxic T cell (CTL) epitopes using mouse MHC class-I alleles (H-2-Db, H-2-Dd, H-2-Kk, H-2-Kb, H-2-Kd and H-2-Ld) based on Stabilized Matrix Method (SMM) [43] and percentile rank ≤ 1 and half-maximal inhibitory concentration of a biological substance $IC_{50} < 500$ nm. Likewise, MHC II binding prediction tools (http://tools.iedb.org/mhcii/) [44] were used to predict helper T-cell (HTL) epitopes. The percentile rank for strong binding peptides was set at ≤ 10 and $IC_{50} < 5000$ nm to determine the interaction potentials of helper T-cell

9

epitope peptide using mouse MHC class II alleles (H2-IAb, H2-IAd and H2-IEd) and based on Stabilized Matrix Method (SMM). The predicted T cell epitopes were classified into high affinity (IC50<50) intermediate affinity (IC50<500) and low affinity (IC50<5000) in binding with mouse MHC alleles.

Visualization of 3D Structures modeling for selected Predicted Epitopes

For protein structure; the secondary structures of predicted amino acids were obtained from Protein Homology/analogY Recognition Engine V 2.0 (phyre2) server (http://www.sbg.bio.ic.ac.uk/phyre2) [45]. The tertiary predicted model of protein was done using UCSF Chimera visualization tool 1.8[46] to visualize and confirm the predicted B and T cell epitopes.

RESULTS

Phylogenetic Analysis of Retrieved Strains

The relationships of all retrieved strains of M polyprotien sequence are illustrated in Figure (1) below.

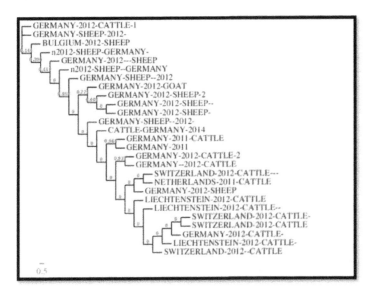

Figure (1): Phylogenetic tree of thr retrived sequences M polyprotien of SBV. (The branch length is proportional to the number of substitutions per site).

Prediction of B-cell epitope and Modeling

M polyprotein (glycoprotein Gn/Gc) sequence was subjected to Bepipred linear epitope prediction, Emini surface accessibility, Kolaskar and Tongaonkar antigenicity, Parker hydrophobicity and Chou and Fasman beta turn prediction methods in IEDB with default thresholds setting. Only one epitope was found to have cutoff prediction scores above threshold scores, namely **QQQACSS** from 764 to 770 in Glycoprotein Gn region, Figure (2). The other epitopes had not satisfied the threshold values of other scales especially Kolaskar and Tongaonkar antigenicity value. The result of all conserved predicted B cell epitopes are listed in Table (3).

11

Table (3): list of B- cell epitopes predicted by different scales for M poly- and NSs protein

Protein type	Bepipred epitope/Threshold0.35	Position	Length	Emini Score	Surface Score	Antigenicity Score	Hydrophilicity Score	Beta Score	Turn	Region
M polyprotein	KEGTRG	21-26	6	2.532		0.885	5.717	1.13		G2
	AEHYKSG	61-67	7	2.111		1	4	1.07		G2
	PIYDD	90-94	5	1.552		1.022	2.44	1.21		G2
	KD	126-127	2	2.133		0.898	7.85	1.235		G2
	TNC	271-273	3	0.637		1.032	4.533	1.237		G2
	KALP	302-305	4	1.056		1.077	0.175	0.945		G2
	*QQQACSS	764-770	7	1.078		1.078	4.929	1.093		G1
	GDKVSNG	932-938	7	1.116		0.959	5.271	1.297		G1
	AMPN	961-964	4	1.019		0.933	1.75	1.085		G1
	KERSSNWGC	1023-1031	9	1.52		0.959	3.867	1.203		G1
	SIEQ	1063-1066	4	1.155		1.007	3.075	0.905		G1
	NDLGSTAKKC	1124-1133	10	1.036		1.002	4.01	1.143		G1
	YNAYSTQ	1216-1222	7	2.851		1.014	3.286	1.124		G1
	PMQSE	1273-1277	5	2.015		0.954	3.64	1.054		G1
	SAYTKPSISK	1299-1310	10	2.69		1.025	3.04	1.106		G1
	TSYIEQHDKK	1321-1330	10	6.536		0.993	3.91	1.015		G1
NSs protein	SSSTRRRP	35-42	8	4.812		0.954	4.925	1.202		-

G1: Glycoprotein Gn G2: Glycoprotein Gc * proposed Epitope. **M polyprotein Threshold:** Emini Surface: 1.000, Antigenicity: 1.039, Hydrophilicity: 0.999 and Beta Turn: 0.986. **NSs protein Threshold:** Emini Surface: 1.000, Antigenicity: 1.029, Hydrophilicity: 0.353 and Beta Turn: 0.981.

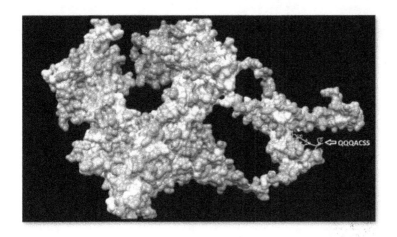

Figure (2): proposed B-Cell Epitope of M polyprotein

Prediction of Cytotoxic T-lymphocyte epitope and interaction with Mouse MHC Class I and Modeling

M polyprotein (glycoprotein Gn/Gc) was analyzed using IEDB MHC-1 binding prediction tool to predict T cell epitope interaction with different types of mouse MHC Class I alleles. 16 peptides had interacted with different mouse MHC-1 alleles. The peptide **YMYNKYFKL** from 251 to 259 in Glycoprotein Gc region had high affinity to interact with one mouse allele (H-2-Kb) $IC_{50}=19.02$ nm and intermediate affinity to bind with H-2-Ld ($IC_{50}=157.34$ nm), followed by **SECCVKDDI** from 46 to 54 and **IVYVFIPIF** from 234 Gc to 242 54 in Glyco-protein Gn which they high affinity to interact with H-2-Kk (IC50=40.03) and H-2-Kb (IC50=40.84) respectively, (Figure 3). The epitopes and their corresponding mouse MHC-1 alleles are shown in Table (4)

Table (4): list of the CTL epitopes which had high and intermediate binding affinity with the mouse MHC Class I alleles in M polyprotein

CTL epitope	Allele	Position	length	percen-tile_rank	SMM IC50(nM)	Region
*YMYNKYFKL	H-2-Kb	251-259	9	0.15	19.02	G2
	H-2-Ld	251-259	9	0.75	157.34	G2
*IVYVFIPIF	H-2-Kb	234-242	9	0.2	40.84	G2
LTMHYFKPL	H-2-Kb	907-915	9	0.25	97.75	G1
YSIKLNCPL	H-2-Db	1278-1286	9	0.3	181.39	G1
*SECCVKDDI	H-2-Kk	46-54	9	0.4	40.03	G2
YIAALQSDI	H-2-Kd	895-903	9	0.5	50.03	G1
YAYMYNKYF	H-2-Kb	249-257	9	0.6	230.2	G2
KPLKNLPAI	H-2-Ld	913-921	9	0.65	199.91	G1
	H-2-Db	913-921	9	0.9	732.18	G1
IKYYRLYQV	H-2-Kb	74-82	9	0.65	167.54	G2
FIPIFYPFV	H-2-Kb	238-246	9	0.7	248.38	G2
VLISNLACL	H-2-Db	6-14	9	0.7	396.84	G2
MMILTKTYI	H-2-Db	226-234	9	0.7	534.1	G2
	H-2-Kd	226-234	9	0.9	906.28	G2
SDIANDLTM	H-2-Db	901-909	9	0.7	221.63	G1

14

TMTLNGDKV	H-2-Db	927-935	9	0.8	651.06	G1
SFCTNLELI	H-2-Db	205-213	9	0.9	210.19	G2
VFIPIFYPF	H-2-Ld	237-245	9	1	226.9	G2

$IC_{50}<50$: High affinity, $Ic_{50}<500$: Intermediate affinity, G1: Glycoprotein Gn, G2: Glycoprotein Gc * proposed Epitope

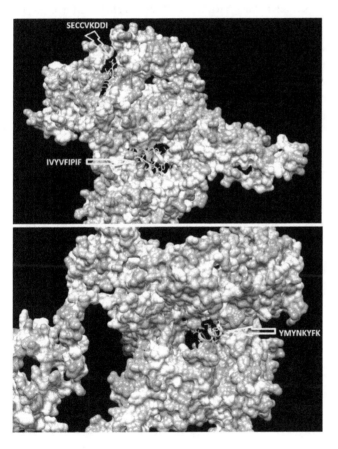

Figure (3): proposed CTL Epitopes of M polyprotein

Prediction of T helper cell epitope and interaction with Mouse MHC Class II and modeling

T-cell epitopes from M polyprotein (glycoprotein Gn/Gc) were predicted using MHC-II binding prediction method. 29 predicted conserved HTL epitopes found to interact with mouse MHC-II alleles (H2-IAb and H2-IAd). The 9-mer peptide (core) **SAYTKPSIS** and **YIE-SHIPAI** in Glycoprotein Gn region had intermediate affinity to interact with H2-IAb allele (IC50= 323 and 464, respectively). While **YRISGTMHV** and **NHYRISGTM** in Glycoprotein Gc region had intermediate affinity to interact with H2-IAb allele (IC50= 490and 497, respectively). The other predicted HTL Epitope had low affinity with these two mice alleles. The result is listed in Table (5) below.

There were several overlaps between MHC Class I epitopes and MHC Class II epitopes. These overlaps are illustrated in Table (6).

Table (5): list of the HTL epitopes which had intermediate and low binding affinity with the mouse MHC Class II alleles in M poly- and NSs protein

Protein type	HTL Epitope (core)	allele	peptide	position	SMM IC50(nM)	Region
M polyprotein	*SAYTKPSIS	H2-IAb	CSASAYTKPSISKNQ	1296-1310	323	G1
	*YIESHIPAI	H2-IAb	RNSYIESHIPAINGL	940-954	464	G1
	*YRISGTMHV	H2-IAb	YRINHYRISGTMHVS	136-150	490	G2
	*NHYRISGTM	H2-IAb	SYRINHYRISGTMHV	135-149	497	G2
	IRNSYIESH	H2-IAb	NGIRNSYIESHIPAI	937-951	524	G1
	FDYNAYSTQ	H2-IAb	MLGDFDYNAYSTQAT	1210-1224	551	G1
	YAFRSSSCS	H2-IAb	LDLRYAFRSSSCSDI	858-872	566	G1
	MHYFKPLKN	H2-IAb	LTMHYFKPLKNLPAI	907-921	687	G1
	FKPLKNLPA	H2-IAb	TMHYFKPLKNLPAII	908-922	917	G1
	LLAVHPFTN	H2-IAb	NCLLAVHPFTNCPST	262-276	1266	G2
	MMMILTKTY	H2-IAd	GSVMMMILTKTYIVY	222-236	1319	G1
	IAALQSDIA	H2-IAd	ENYIAALQSDIANDL	893-907	1414	G1
	VMMMILTKT	H2-IAd	ILVGSVMMMILTKTY	219-233	1580	G2
	VHPFTNCPS	H2-IAb	LLAVHPFTNCPSTCI	264-278	1861	G2
	TIYIIISLI	H2-IAd	YWRLTIYIIISLIML	1357-1371	1868	G1
	YIKIIAVDP	H2-IAd	DTYIKIIAVDPMQSE	1263-1277	1917	G1
	MILTKTYIV	H2-IAd	VMMMILTKTYIVYVF	224-238	2149	G2

17

MYKWPSLGV	H2-IAd	KSKMYKWPSLGVYKH	746-760	2369	G1
TSHMEVHKK	H2-IAd	ASTSHMEVHKKVSSV	1188-1202	2986	G1
IKIIAVDPM	H2-IAd	TYIKIIAVDPMQSEY	1264-1278	3146	G1
VDPMQSEYS	H2-IAd	IKIIAVDPMQSEYSI	1266-1280	3719	G1
MEVHKKVSS	H2-IAd	STSHMEVHKKVSSVG	1189-1203	3839	G1
SIKLNCPLA	H2-IAd	MQSEYSIKLNCPLAT	1274-188	4545	G1
QLDIQTIQM	H2-IAd	DRIQLDIQTIQMDSM	1093-1107	4594	G1
LYQVKDWHS	H2-IAd	IKYYRLYQVKDWHSC	74-88	4880	G2
YRLYQVKDW	H2-IAd	VIKYYRLYQVKDWHS	73-87	4884	G2
YTTTESLKL	H2-IAd	IYTTTESLKLHRMCN	282-294	4905	G2
DRIQLDIQT	H2-IAd	PLISDRIQLDIQTIQ	1089-1103	7382	G1
IKYYRLYQV	H2-IAd	RLAAVIKYYRLYQVK	69-83	8525	G2
STRRPRWS	H2-IEd	SSSTRRRPRWSYIRR	35-49	727	-
SSSTRRRPR	H2-IEd	ESSSSTRRRPRWSYI	33-47	1890	-
RRPRWSYIR	H2-IAd	TRRRPRWSYIRRHNQ	38-52	3104	-

NSs protein

IC_{50}<500: Intermediate affinity, Ic_{50}<5000: Low affinity, G1: Glycoprotein Gn, G2: Glycoprotein Gc *proposed Epitope

18

Table (6): Overlapping between MHC class I and II T cell epitopes in M polyprotein

HTL Epitopes	allele	peptide	Position	Region	CTL Epitopes
MHYFKPLKN	H2-IAb	**LTMHYFKPL**KNLPAI	907-921	G1	LTMHYFKPL
	H2-IAb	LTMHYF**KPLKNLPAI**	907-921	G1	KPLKNLPAI
FKPLKNLPA	H2-IAb	TMHYF**KPLKNLPAI**I	908-922	G1	
MMMILTKTY	H2-IAd	GSVM**MMILTKTYI**VY	222-236	G2	MMILTKTYI
IAALQSDIA	H2-IAd	ENY**IAALQSDI**ANDL	893-907	G1	YIAALQSDI
MILTKTYIV	H2-IAd	V**MMMILTKTYIVY**VF	224-238	G2	MMILTKTYI
SIKLNCPLA	H2-IAd	MQSE**YSIKLNCPL**AT	1274-1288	G1	YSIKLNCPL
LYQVKDWHS	H2-IAd	**IKYYRLYQV**KDWHSC	74-88	G2	IKYYRLYQV
YRLYQVKDW	H2-IAd	V**IKYYRLYQV**KDWHS	73-87	G2	

The underlined and highlighted residues are the 9-mer MHC class I T cell epitopes overlapping the 15-mer MHC class II T cell epitopes. G1: Glycoprotein Gn, G2: Glycoprotein Gc

DISCUSSION

SBV can cause considerable economic loss [47,48]. Unfortunately there is no treatment or vaccine for animals infected with the Schmallenberg virus [49]. Vaccination against SBV could play an important role in disease control. So; in this study we aimed to determine the highly potential immunogenic epitopes for B and T cells as vaccine candidate for M polyprotein (glycoprotein Gn/Gc) and NSs protein in Schmallenberg virus.

In this study, we excluded the NSm in M polyprotein segment because this part is not important for viral replication, in contrast with NSs protein in S segment contributes to viral pathogenesis by blocking the production of interferon (IFN) leading to inhibition the innate responses of the host [50]. We focused on the envelope glycoproteins Gn and Gc regions on M polyprotein also, because these regions have essential role for viral attachment and cell fusion [6-8] and can be recognized by neutralizing antibodies [51].

As we all know; B cell epitopes may be linear (continuous) or conformational (discontinuous). The protective linear B-cell epitopes may lead to the synthesis of the efficient peptide vaccine against viral disease [52]. Based on this fact; we chose our predicted B cell epitopes to be linear (continuous). To determine a potential and effective epitopes for B cell, predicted epitopes should get above threshold scores in Bepipred linear epitope prediction, Emini surface accessibility, Parker hydrophilicity, Kolaskar and Tongaonkar antigenicity and Chou and Fasman beta turn prediction methods in IEDB. As the results illustrated in Table (3); we found [764]QQQACSS[770] epitope in Glycoprotein Gn region of M polyprotein was the only epitope that had cutoff prediction scores above threshold scores. We predicted only one conserved epitope In NSs region namely [35]SSSTRRRP[42] and we found that this epitope had satisfied all scales except antigenicity test.

Designing vaccine against T cell epitope is much more promising due to long lasting immune response and antigenic drift where antigen can easily escape the antibody memory response [53]. We used mouse MHC alleles to identify epitopes in a cattle, goat and sheep study, based on Gurung R.B. et.al. (2012) study where they found more than 80% identity between the MHC alleles of mice, sheep, and cow. In addition, bovine MHC profile in particular is more complex than the mouse MHC profile [54]. In our study; we found three CTL Epitopes in Gly-

20

coprotein GC region namely ^{251}**YMYNKYFKL**^{259}, ^{46}**SECCVKDDI**^{54} and ^{234}**IVYVFIPIF**^{242} had high affinity to interact with one mouse allele. We did not predict any promising CTL epitopes in NSs region against SBV.

According to Table (5); we found four 9-mer HTL epitopes (core) interacted with mouse MHC-II alleles (H2-IAb and H2-IAd) namely ^{1299}**SAYTKPSIS**^{1307} and ^{943}**YIESHIPAI**^{951} in Glycoprotein Gn region and ^{140}**YRISGTMHV**^{149} and ^{139}**NHYRISGTM**^{147} in Glycoprotein Gc region but we found that their bindings were intermediate affinity. While three epitopes were predicted in NSs region **STRRRPRWS**, **SSSTRRRPR** and **RRPRWSYIR** but their affinities were low. Also we found ^{74}**IKYYRLYQV**^{82} epitope was common in both MHC class I and II.

Our results represented in Table (6). We observed several Overlaps between MHC class I and II T cell epitopes in M polyprotein. We expected these overlaps suggest the possibility of antigen presentation to immune cells via both MHC class I and II pathways.

In summary; after screening the epitopes; it was clear that Glycoprotein regions (Gn and Gc) of M polyprotein in SBV can be used for the preparation of immunological constructs. Our studies suggested that; B cell epitope ^{764}**QQQACSS**^{770} and CTL epitopes ^{251}**YMYNKYFKL**^{259}, ^{46}**SECCVKDDI**^{54} and ^{234}**IVYVFIPIF**^{242} can be used as a potential vaccine candidate against SBV.

CONCLUSION

Our study involved the usage of peptide vaccine strategy based on the predictive and analytic tool (IEDB-AR). This strategy is the up-to-date approach to develop vaccines. Also it depends on the usage of short peptide fragments (epitopes) contained within single protein of the microbes to induce positive, desirable T- and B-cell mediated immune responses. In addition, peptide vaccines have the advantage of the exclusion of unnecessary antigenic load and does not induce immune response. We can confirm our findings by adding complementary steps of both in vitro and in vivo studies to support this new universal predicted vaccine for ruminants against SBV.

Acknowledgments

Authors would like to thanks African City of Technology members for their assistance and help.

Competing Interests

The authors declare that they have no competing interests.

References

1. Lazutka J, Zvirbliene A, Dalgediene I, Petraityte-Burneikiene R, Spakova A, Sereika V. *et. al*. Generation of Recombinant Schmallenberg Virus Nucleocapsid Protein in Yeast and Development of Virus-Specific Monoclonal Antibodies. *Journal of Immunology Research* 2014; 2014. Available at http://dx.doi.org/10.1155/2014/160316

2. Doceul V, Lara E, Sailleau C, Belbis G, Richardson J, Bréard E. *et. al*. Epidemiology, molecular virology and diagnostics of Schmallenberg virus, an emerging orthobunyavirus in Europe.*Veterinary Research*. 2013; 44:31. DOI: 10.1186/1297-9716-44-31

3. Hechinger S, Wernike K, Beer M. Evaluating the protective efficacy of a trivalent vaccine containing Akabane virus, Aino virus and Chuzan virus against Schmallenberg virus infection. *Vet Res.*2013; 44(1):114. DOI: 10.1186/1297-9716-44-1141.

4. Hover S, King B, Hall B, Loundras EA, Taqi H, Daly J, et. al. Modulation of Potassium Channels Inhibits Bunyavirus Infection. Biological chemistry 2016;291(7):3411–3422. DOI: 10.1074/jbc.M115.692673jbc.M115.692673.

5. Poskin A, Verite S, Comtet L, Stede Y, Cay B, Regge N. Persistence of the protective immunityand kinetics of the isotype specific antibody response against the viral nucleocapsid protein after experimental Schmallenberg virus infection of sheep. Veterinary research. 2015;46:119. DOI:10.1186/s13567-015-0260-6

6. Varela M, Pinto RM, Caporale M, Piras IM, Taggart A, Seehusen F. *et. al*. Mutations in the Schmallenberg Virus Gc Glycoprotein Facilitate Cellular Protein Synthesis Shutoff and Restore Pathogenicity of NSs Deletion Mutants in Mice. *J Virol* 2016; 90 (11):5440-50. DOI: 10.1128/JVI.00424-16.

7. Blomström AL, Gu Q, Barry G, Wilkie G, Skelton JK, Baird M. *e.t al.* Transcriptome analysis reveals the host response to Schmallenberg virus in bovine cells and antagonistic effects of the NSs protein. BMC Genomics 2015; 16:324. DOI: 10.1186/s12864-015-1538-9

8. Wernike K, Brocchi E, Cordioli P, Sénéchal Y, Schelp C, Wegelt A. *et. al.* A novel panel of monoclonal antibodies against Schmallenberg virus nucleoprotein and glycoprotein Gc allows specific orthobunyavirus detection and reveals antigenic differences. Veterinary Research 2015; 46:27. DOI: 10.1186/s13567-015-0165-4

9. Fieke M. Molenaar, S. Anna La Rocca, Meenakshi Khatri, Javier Lopez, Falko Steinbach, Akbar Dastjerdi. Exposure of Asian Elephants and Other Exotic Ungulates to Schmallenberg Virus. *PLoS ONE* 2015; 10(8): e0135532. **DOI:**10.1371/journal.pone.0135532

10. Mouchantat S, Wernike K, Lutz W, Hoffmann B, Ulrich RG, Börner K, Wittstatt U, Beer M. A broad spectrum screening of Schmallenberg virus antibodies in wildlife animals in Germany. Veterinary Research. 2015; 46:99. DOI: 10.1186/s13567-015-0232-x

11. Jon Wensman JJ, Blomqvist G, Hjort M, Holst BS. Presence of Antibodies to Schmallenberg Virus in a Dog in Sweden. Jour*nal of Clinical Microbiology* 2013, 51 (8):2802–2803. DOI:10.1128/JCM.00877-13

12. Manley R, Harrup LE, Veronesi E, Stubbins F, Stoner J, Gubbins S, *et. al.* Testing of UK Populations of Culex pipiens L. for Schmallenberg Virus Vector Competence and Their Colonization. *PLoS ONE* 2015; 10(8):e0134453. DOI:10.1371/journal. pone.0134453

13. Kluiters G, Pagès N, Carpenter S, Gardès L, Guis H, Baylis M, Garros C. Morphometric discrimination of two sympatric sibling species in the Palaearctic region, Culicoides obsoletus Meigen and C. scoticus Downes & Kettle (Diptera: Ceratopogonidae), vectors of bluetongue and Schmallenberg viruses. *Parasites & Vectors* 2016; 9(1):262. DOI 10.1186/s13071-016-1520-7.

14. Ponsart C, Pozzi N, Bréard E, Catinot V, Viard G, Sailleau C. *et. al.* Evidence of excretion of Schmallenberg virus in bull semen *Veterinary Research* 2014; 45:37. DOI: 10.1186/1297-9716-45-37.

15. Varela M, Schnettler E, Caporale M, Murgia C, Barry G, McFarlane M, *.e.t al.* Schmallenberg Virus Pathogenesis, Tropism and Interaction with the Innate Immune System of the Host *.PLoS Pathog.* 2013; 9(1):e1003133. DOI:10.1371/journal.ppat.1003133

16. Martinelle L, Poskin A, Dal Pozzo F, De Regge N, Cay B, Saegerman. Experimental Infection of Sheep at 45 and 60 Days of Gestation with Schmallenberg Virus Readily Led to Placental Colonization without Causing Congenital Malformations. *PLoS ONE 2015;* 10(9): e0139375. DOI:10.1371/journal.pone.0139375

17. Wernike K, Holsteg M, Schirrmeier H, Hoffmann B, Beer M. Natural Infection of Pregnant Cows with Schmallenberg Virus – A Follow-Up Study. *PLoS ONE* 2014; 9(5): e98223. DOI:10.1371/journal.pone.0098223

18. Herder V, Hansmann F, Wohlsein P, Peters M, Varela M, Palmarini M, *et al.* Immunophenotyping of Inflammatory Cells Associated with Schmallenberg Virus Infection of the Central Nervous System of Ruminants . *PLoS ONE* 2013; 8(5): e62939. DOI:10.1371/journal.pone.0062939

19. Barrett DJ, More SJ, O'Neill RG, Collins DM, O'Keefe C, Regazzoli V, Sammin D. Short communication:Exposure to Schmallenberg virus in Irish sheep in 2013. *Veterinary Record* 2015; 177(19):494. DOI: 10.1136/vr.103318

20. Harris KA, Eglin RD, Hayward S, Milnes A, Davies I, Cook AJ, Downs SH. Paper:Impact of Schmallenberg virus on British sheep farms during the 2011/2012 lambing season. *Veterinary Record* 2014;176246. DOI: 10.1136/vr.102295

21. Monaco F, Goffredo M, Federici V, Carvelli A, Capobianco Dondona A, Polci A, Pinoni C, Danzetta ML, Selli L, Bonci M, Quaglia M, Calistri P. First cases of Schmallenberg virus in Italy: surveillance strategies. *Vet Ital.* 2013; 49(3): 269-275. DOI:10.12834/VetIt.1101.11

22. Blomström AL, Stenberg H, Scharin I, Figueiredo J, Nhambirre O, Abilio AP, Fafetine J, Berg M. Serological Screening Suggests Presence of Schmallenberg Virus in Cattle, Sheep and Goat in the Zambezia Province, Mozambique. *Transbound Emerg Dis.* 2014; 61(4):289–292. DOI: 10.1111/tbed.12234.

23. Paul R. Bessell, Harriet K. Auty, Kate R. Searle, Ian G. Handel, Bethan V. Purse & B. Mark de C. Bronsvoort. *Scientific Reports.* Impact of temperature, feeding preference and vaccination on Schmallenberg virus transmission in Scotland. Scientific Reports. 2014; 5746(4). DOI: 10.1038/srep05746

24. Luttikholt S, Veldhuis A, van den Brom R, Moll L, Lievaart-Peterson K, Peperkamp K, et al. Risk Factors for Malformations and Impact on Reproductive Performance and Mortality Rates of Schmallenberg Virus in Sheep Flocks in the Netherlands. PLoS ONE 2014; 9(6): e100135. DOI:10.1371/journal.pone.0100135

25. Barrett D, More SJ, O'Neill R, Bradshaw B, Casey M, Keane M, McGrath G, Sammin D. Prevalence and distribution of exposure to Schmallenberg virus in Irish cattle during October 2012 to November 2013. BMC Vet Res. 2015; 11: 267. DOI:10.1186/s12917-015-0564-9

26. Larska M, Krzysiak MK, Kęsik-Maliszewska J, Rola J. Cross-sectional study of Schmallenberg virus seroprevalence in wild ruminants in Poland at the end of the vector season of 2013. *BMC Vet Res.* 2014; 10:967. DOI 10.1186/s12917-014-0307-3

27. Dominguez M., Gache K., Touratier A,. Perrin J.B., Fediaevsky A., Collin E., Bréard E. *et. al.* Spread and impact of the Schmallenberg virus epidemic in France in 2012-2013. *BMC Veterinary Research* 2014; 10:248.

28. Kraatz F, Wernike K, Hechinger S, König P, Granzow H, Reimann I, Beer M. Deletion mutants of Schmallenberg virus are avirulent and protect from virus challenge. *J Virol* 2015; 89:1825–1837. DOI:10.1128/JVI.02729-14.

29. Wernike K, Nikolin VM, Hechinger S, Hoffmann B, Beer M. Inactivated Schmallenberg virus prototype vaccines. *Vaccine* 2013; 31 (35):3558-63. DOI:10.1016/j.vaccine.2013.05.062

.

30. Hechinger S., Wernike K., Beer M. Single immunization with an inactivated vaccine protects sheep from Schmallenberg virus Infection. *Veterinary Research* 2014;45:79. DOI: 10.1186/s13567-014-0079-6.

31. Johnson A, Bradshaw B, Boland C, Ross P. A bulk milk tank study to detect evidence of spread of Schmallenberg virus infection in the south west of Ireland in 2013. *Irish Veterinary Journal* 2014; 67:11. DOI: 10.1186/2046-0481-67-11

32. Mellor PS, Boorman J, Baylis M. Culicoides biting midges: their role as arbovirus vectors. *Annu Rev Entomol* 2000;45 :307–40. [PMID: 10761580] DOI: 10.1146/annurev.ento.45.1.307

33. Zientara S, MacLachlan NJ, Calistri P, Sanchez-Vizcaino JM, Savini G. Bluetongue vaccination in Europe. *Expert Rev Vaccines* 2010; 9(9): 989–91. DOI: 10.1586/erv.10.97.

34. Dereeper A., Guignon V., Blanc G., Audic S., Buffet S., Chevenet F., Dufayard J.F., Guindon S., Lefort V., Lescot M., Claverie J.M., Gascuel O. Phylogeny.fr: robust phylogenetic analysis for the non-specialist. *Nucleic Acids Res.* 2008; (Web Server issue):W465-9. [PMID: 18424797]

35. Tom H. BioEdit: An important software for molecular biology. *GERF Bulletin of Biosciences.* 2011; 2(1): 60-61

36. Bui H. H,Sidney J, Li W, Fusseder N, Sette A. Development of an epitope conservancy analysis tool to facilitate the design of epitope-based diagnostics and vaccines. *BMC Bioinformatics.*2007; 8(1):361. PMID: 17897458

37. Vita R, Overton JA, Greenbaum JA, Ponomarenko J, Clark JD, Cantrell JR, Wheeler DK, Gabbard JL, Hix D, Sette A, Peters B. The immune epitope database (IEDB) 3.0. *Nucleic Acids Res.* 2014 Oct 9. pii: gku938. [Epub ahead of print] PubMed PMID: 25300482.

38. Larsen JE, Lund O, Nielsen M. Improved method for predicting linear B-cell epitopes. *ImmunomeRes.*2006;2:2 PMID: 16635264

39. Emini EA, Hughes JV, Perlow DS, Boger J. Induction of hepatitis A virus-neutralizing antibody by a virus-specific synthetic peptide. *J Virol*. 1985; 55(3):836-9. PMID: 2991600

40. Kolaskar AS, Tongaonkar PC. A semi-empirical method for prediction of antigenic determinants on protein antigens. *FEBS Lett*. 1990; 276(1-2):172-4. PMID: 1702393

41. Parker JM, Guo D, Hodges RS. New hydrophilicity scale derived from high-performance liquid chromatography peptide retention data: correlation of predicted surface residues with antigenicity and X-ray-derived accessible sites. *Biochemistry*. 1986; 25(19):5425-32. PMID: 2430611

42. Chou PY, Fasman GD. Prediction of the secondary structure of proteins from their amino acid sequence. *Adv Enzymol Relat Areas Mol Biol*.1978; 47:45-148. PMID: 364941

43. Peters B, Sette A. Generating quantitative models describing the sequence specificity of biological processes with the stabilized matrix method. *BMC Bioinformatics* 2005; 6:132. PMID: 15927070

44. Wang P, Sidney J, Kim Y, Sette A, Lund O, Nielsen M, Peters B. Peptide binding predictions for HLA DR, DP and DQ molecules. *BMC Bioinformatics*.2010;11:568. PMID: 21092157

45. Kelley LA, Mezulis S., Yates CM., Wass MN. , Sternberg MJ. The Phyre2 web portal for protein modeling, prediction and analysis. *Nature Protocols* 2015; (10): 845-858. *DOI*:10.1038/nprot.2015.05

46. Pettersen EF, Goddard TD, Huang CC, Couch GS, Greenblatt DM, Meng EC, Ferrin TE. UCSF Chimera--a visualization system for exploratory research and analysis. *J Comput Chem*. 2004;25(13):1605-12. PMID:15264254

47. Martinelle L, Dal Pozzo F, Gauthier B, Kirschvink N, Saegerman C. Field veterinary survey on clinical and economic impact of Schmallenberg virus in Belgium. *Transbound Emerg Dis*. 2014 ;61(3):285-8. DOI:10.1111/tbed.12030

48. Dominguez M, Hendrikx P, Zientara S, Calavas D, Jay M, Touratier A, et al. Preliminary estimate of Schmallenberg virus infection impact in sheep flocks – France. *Vet Rec*. 2012;171 (17):426. DOI: 10.1136/vr.100883.

49. Wernike K, Nikolin VM, Hechinger S, Hoffmann B, Beer M. Inactivated Schmallenberg virus prototype vaccines. *Vaccine.* 2013; 31(35): 3558–63. DOI: 10.1016/j.vaccine.2013.05.062.

50. Varela M, Schnettler E, Caporale M, Murgia C, Barry G, McFarlane M, *et al.* Schmallenberg Virus Pathogenesis, Tropism and Interaction with the Innate Immune System of the Host. *PLoS Pathog* 2013; 9(1): e1003133. DOI:10.1371/journal.ppat.1003133

51. Pawaiya RV, Gupta VK. A review on Schmallenberg virus infection: a newly emerging disease of cattle, sheep and goats. *Veterinarni Medicina.* 2013; 58(10):516-26.

52. Saha S., Raghava G.P.S. Prediction of Continuous B-Cell Epitopes in an Antigen Using Recurrent Neural Network. *PROTEINS: Structure, Function, and Bioinformatics* 2006; 65:40–48. DOI: 10.1002/prot.21078

53. Shawan MM, Mahmud HA, Hasan M, Parvin A, Rahman M, Rahman SM.. In Silico Modeling and Immunoinformatics Probing Disclose the Epitope Based PeptideVaccine Against. Zika Virus Envelope Glycoprotein. *Indian J. Pharm. Biol. Res.* 2014; 2(4):44-57.

54. Ratna B. Gurung, Auriol C. Purdie, Douglas J. Begg and Richard J. Whittington. In Silico Identification of Epitopes in Mycobacterium avium subsp.paratuberculosis Proteins That Were Upregulated under Stress Condition. *Clin. Vaccine Immunol.* 2012, 19(6):855. DOI:10.1128/CVI.00114-12.s

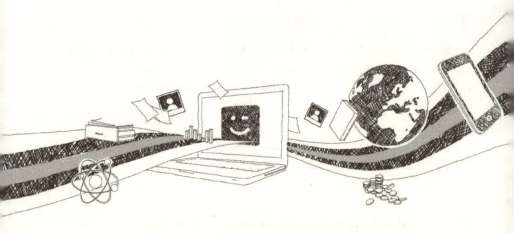
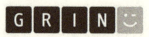